1

Table of Contents

PREVIEW

Cirrhosis is a late-stage liver disease in which healthy liver tissue is replaced with scar tissue and the liver is permanently damaged. Scar tissue keeps your liver from working properly.

Many types of liver diseases and conditions injure healthy liver cells, causing cell death and inflammation. This is followed by cell repair and finally tissue scarring as a result of the repair process.

The scar tissue blocks the flow of blood through the liver and slows the liver's ability to process nutrients, hormones, drugs and natural toxins (poisons). It also reduces the production of proteins and other substances made by the liver. Cirrhosis eventually keeps the liver from working properly. Late-stage cirrhosis is life-threatening.

CIRRHOSIS DIET RECIPES

BREAKFAST

Prep Time: 10 Minutes

Cook Time: 30 Minutes

Servings: 2

Ingredients

- 2 tsp dark sesame oil
- 1 clove garlic (minced)
- 2 tsp fresh ginger (peeled and minced)
- 1 small onion (diced)
- 1/4 large red bell pepper (diced)
- 12 ounces Yukon Gold potatoes (large dice)
- 2 tsp low sodium soy sauce or gluten-free tamari sauce
- fresh ground black pepper to taste

Instructions

1. Place the oil in a skillet over medium heat. Add the garlic and ginger and sauté for about 2 minutes. Stir frequently. Add the onions and sauté, stirring frequently, for about 3 minutes or until translucent. Add the bell pepper and continue sautéing for 2 minutes.

   Add the potatoes, stir, and cover. Reduce heat to medium and cook for about 15 minutes, stirring frequently, until the potatoes are soft.

   Add the soy sauce and pepper and stir. Cook for another 5 minutes on low. Serve.

Prep Time: 10 Minutes

Cook Time: 40 Minutes

Servings: 2

Ingredients

- 2 tsp. olive oil
- 2 large shallots (thinly sliced)
- 1 small avocado
- 1/16 tsp. salt
- ground black pepper to taste
- 1/4 lemon (juiced)
- 1 ounce feta cheese (crumbled)
- 2 slices whole grain or gluten free bread

Instructions

2. Place a small skillet over medium.
3. When the skillet is hot add the oil to the pan and swirl to coat.
4. Add the shallots and toss to coat well. Sauté for about 10 minutes until caramelized.

5. Adjust the heat so that the shallots brown but do not burn.

6. When the shallots are cooked, set aside.

7. While the shallots are roasting, mash the avocado in a small bowl.

8. Add the salt, pepper, and lemon juice, and fold together.

9. Toast the bread and then spread the avocado mixture on top.

10. Top with the caramelized shallot and then the crumbled feta.

11. Serve.

Prep Time: 10 Minutes

Cook Time: 40 Minutes

Servings: 2

Ingredients

- 1 tsp. olive oil
- 4 ounces cherry or grape tomatoes
- 1 large shallot (thinly sliced)
- 1 small avocado
- 1/16 tsp. salt
- ground black pepper to taste
- 1/4 lemon (juiced)
- 2 tsp. capers
- 2 slices whole grain or gluten free bread
- 4 large leaves fresh basil (chiffonade)

Instructions

1. Place a small skillet in the oven and preheat to 350°F.
2. When the oven is hot add the oil to the pan and swirl to coat.

3. Add the tomatoes and shallots and toss to coat well and return the pan to the oven.

4. Roast the tomatoes and shallots for about 10 to 12 minutes. Toss about every 3 to 4 minutes.

5. While the tomatoes and shallots are roasting mash the avocado in a small bowl.

6. Add the salt, pepper and lemon juice and fold together.

7. After the tomatoes and shallots have roasted about 10 to 12 minutes add the capers.

8. Toss and return the pan to the oven for 4 to 5 minutes.

9. Toast the bread and then spread the avocado mixture on top.

10. Top with the roasted shallot, caper, and tomato mixture, then the basil.

11. Serve.

Prep Time: 25 Minutes

Cook Time: 40 Minutes

Servings: 2

Ingredients

- 1/2 cup blue cornmeal
- 1/4 cup whole wheat flour
- 2 tsp Splenda or stevia
- 1 tsp baking powder
- 1/4 tsp salt
- 2/3 cup non-fat buttermilk
- 1 large egg
- 1 tsp pure vanilla extract
- 2 Tbsp (per serving) fresh blueberries
- 2 tsp (per serving) unsalted butter
- 1 Tbsp pure maple syrup

Instructions

1. Place the blue cornmeal, whole wheat flour, Splenda, baking powder and salt in a sifter and sift into a

medium sized mixing bowl. Add the buttermilk, egg, and vanilla extract and whisk until smooth. Heat a non-stick griddle over medium-high heat. Let the batter stand for at least 2 minutes while the griddle is heating. Stir once and wait another minute before placing batter on the griddle. When the griddle is hot enough that a few drops of water will sputter on the surface, reduce the heat to medium and place about 1/4 cup of batter for each pancake on the griddle. After the pancakes have cooked for about a minute spread a tablespoon of blueberries across the top of each one. Allow to cook for another 1 - 2 minutes until bubbles form on the surface and burst. Turn pancake and cook for about 1/2 the time of the first side until they are golden brown. Remove and top with one teaspoon of butter on each pancake and serve one tablespoon of pure maple syrup for every two pancakes.

Prep Time: 25 Minutes

Cook Time: 55 Minutes

Servings: 2

Ingredients

- 1 Tbsp. olive oil
- 1 1/2 Tbsp. balsamic vinegar
- 1 tsp. honey
- 1/8 tsp. cayenne pepper
- 1/8 tsp. salt
- 8 ounces crimini mushrooms (quartered)
- 1 clove garlic (finely minced)
- 2 slices whole grain or gluten free bread
- 1 small avocado
- 1/16 tsp. salt
- ground black pepper to taste
- 1/4 lemon (juiced)

Instructions

2. Preheat the oven to 350°F.

3. Place the olive oil, balsamic vinegar, honey, cayenne pepper, and salt in a small roasting pan or large skillet.

4. Whisk together until well blended.

5. Add the mushrooms and garlic and fold together until well coated.

6. Place the pan in the oven and roast for 15 to 20 minutes. Stir every 5 minutes or so.

7. Remove from the oven when the mushrooms are well caramelized.

8. While the mushrooms are roasting, mash the avocado in a small bowl.

9. Add the salt, pepper, and lemon juice and fold together.

10. When the mushrooms are cooked, toast the bread and then spread the avocado mixture on top.

11. Top with the balsamic mushrooms and serve.

Prep Time: 15 Minutes

Cook Time: 35 Minutes

Servings: 2

Ingredients

- 1 tsp. olive oil
- 1 large shallot (finely diced)
- 1 cup no salt added black beans (drained and rinsed)
- 1/4 tsp. ground cumin
- 1 tsp. smoked paprika
- 1/2 tsp. dried oregano leaves
- 1/2 cup water
- 1 small avocado
- 1/16 tsp. salt
- ground black pepper to taste
- 1/4 lemon (juiced)
- 2 slices whole grain or gluten free bread

Instructions

1. Place a small skillet over medium.

2. When the pan is hot add the oil to the pan and swirl to coat.

3. Add the shallots and cook for about 2 minutes.

4. Adjust the heat so that the shallots brown but do not burn.

5. Add the black beans, cumin, paprika, oregano and water.

6. Simmer until all of the water has evaporated.

7. Set aside.

8. While the beans are cooking mash the avocado in a small bowl.

9. Add the salt, pepper and lemon juice and fold together.

10. Toast the bread and then spread the avocado mixture on top.

11. Top with the beans.

12. Serve.

Prep Time: 35 Minutes

Cook Time: 1hrs 15 Minutes

Servings: 4

Ingredients

- 1 Tbsp olive oil
- 2 cloves garlic (sliced)
- 1 large onion (diced)
- 1 15 ounce can no salt added crushed tomatoes
- 1 Tbsp chili powder
- 1 tsp ground cumin
- 1 tsp dried oregano
- 1 small chipotle pepper in adobo sauce (optional) (minced)
- 1/4 tsp salt
- fresh ground black pepper to taste
- 5 cups water
- 1 cup brown or green lentils
- 6 Tbsp non-fat sour cream
- 6 ounces reduced-fat Monterey jack cheese (shredded)

Instructions

1. Place the olive oil in a large saucepan, over medium heat.
2. Add the garlic and onion and cook, stirring frequently, until the onions have softened.
3. Add the crushed tomatoes, chili powder, cumin, oregano, chipotle (if used), salt, and pepper, and stir well.
4. Add the water and the lentils, and stir well.
5. Reduce heat to medium-low and simmer until lentils are cooked through but not mushy, approximately 45 minutes to an hour.
6. Serve with 1 1/2 tablespoon sour cream and 1/2 ounce Monterey jack cheese per serving.

Prep Time: 15 Minutes

Cook Time: 35 Minutes

Servings: 2

Ingredients

French Toast:

- 1 large egg
- 2 tsp. Grand Marnier orange liqueur
- 1/2 tsp. sugar
- 1 Tbsp. 2% milk
- 1/4 tsp. pure vanilla extract
- 1/4 cup orange juice
- 1/4 tsp. orange zest
- 4 slices sourdough bread
- 2 tsp. (per serving) unsalted butter

Orange Honey:

- 2 Tbsp. honey
- 1/2 tsp. Grand Marnier orange liqueur

Instructions

1. Place the egg, Grand Marnier, sugar, milk, vanilla extract, orange juice, and orange peel in a medium mixing bowl.
2. Whisk until well blended.
3. Heat a non-stick griddle over medium-high heat.
4. When the griddle is hot enough that a few drops of water will dance on the surface, reduce the heat to medium and place 4 slices of bread into the batter.
5. Gently dunk and turn the bread until it is well coated and slightly soaked.
6. Place the 4 slices of soaked bread on the griddle and cook for about 3 – 4 minutes. Turn and cook on the other side.
7. Cook, turning occasionally, until both sides are golden brown.
8. Depending on your stove or griddle you may need to reduce the heat slightly.
9. Remove and top with the butter and orange honey.

Prep Time: 10 Minutes

Cook Time: 35 Minutes

Servings: 6

Ingredients

- 1 large egg (separated)
- 2 tsp unsalted butter
- 1 large banana
- 1/2 tsp pure vanilla extract
- 1/2 cup Z-Sweet stevia or Splenda
- 1/4 cup chopped pecans
- 1 cup all purpose white flour
- 1/2 cup whole wheat flour
- 2 Tbsp wheat germ
- 1/4 tsp salt
- 1 tsp baking powder
- 1/4 tsp baking soda
- 1/2 tsp ground cinnamon
- 1/4 tsp ground nutmeg
- 1/4 cup low-fat buttermilk
- 2 tsp light brown sugar

Instructions

1. Preheat oven to 375°F. Using a whisk, cream together the egg yolk and light spread. Add the banana and mash into the mixture until well blended. Add the vanilla extract and Splenda and blend. Fold in the chopped pecans. Sift the all purpose flour, whole wheat flour, wheat germ, salt, baking powder, baking soda, cinnamon and nutmeg in a sifter and sift into the mixing bowl.

2. Gently fold the creamed mixture together with the flour mixture until smooth. When blended the mixture will still be dry. Whisk the egg white until it is white and foamy (about tripled in volume). Fold in the egg white. Fold in the buttermilk, and when the dough is just blended together, stop. Line a standard size muffin tin with 6 muffin papers and fill each muffin paper with an equal amount of batter. Sprinkle the brown sugar over the tops of the muffins.

3. Place the muffins in the oven and bake for 20 minutes.

Prep Time: 10 Minutes

Cook Time: 35 Minutes

Servings: 2

Ingredients

- 1 tsp olive oil
- 1/2 medium white onion (minced)
- 2 tsp all purpose flour
- 2 ears fresh corn (cut kernels off cob)
- 1/4 tsp salt
- 1/2 cup 2% milk
- 1 cup water
- fresh ground black pepper to taste

Instructions

1. Heat the canola oil in a medium sized skillet over medium heat. Add the minced onion and cook for about 3 - 5 minutes until they begin to soften.

Add the flour and stir until it is well blended into the onions.

2. Add the corn kernels and cook for about 3 minutes stirring frequently. Add the salt, milk, water and pepper.

   Cook over medium heat simmering for about 20 minutes stirring frequently.

   Remove half of the corn from the pan and place in a blender. Pulse the blender until the corn is smooth.

   Add the mixture back to the skillet with the remaining corn.

   Reheat gently while stirring. Serve.

11. Butternut Squash Tortilla

Prep Time: 10 Minutes

Cook Time: 60 Minutes

Servings: 2

Ingredients

- 1 small butternut squash (about 1 pound)
- 2 tsp olive oil
- 1 large onion (sliced)
- 6 large eggs
- 1/4 tsp salt
- 1 Tbsp water
- 2 ounces prosciutto or other good-quality ham (finely diced)

Instructions

1. Place a large skillet in the oven and preheat the oven to 325°F.

2. Cut the squash in half lengthwise and scoop out the seeds.

3. Place 1 teaspoon of the olive oil in the pan and add the squash, cut side down.

4. Roast for about 45 minutes until very soft.

5. Scoop the flesh from the squash into a large bowl and discard the rind. Mash the squash gently with a fork until it is the consistency of mashed potatoes. Set aside to cool.

6. Place the other teaspoon of olive oil in a 12-inch skillet over medium-high heat and add the onions. Cook, stirring frequently, until limp but not browned.

7. While the onions are cooking, place the eggs and water in a large bowl and whisk until frothy.

8. Add the diced ham to the eggs and whisk until blended.

9. Add the salt and the mashed butternut squash and fold together until just blended. Do not overmix or the squash will become pasty.

10. Reduce the heat beneath the onions to medium and add the squash and egg mixture to the pan. Fold together gently.

11. Place the skillet in the oven and bake for 20 to 25 minutes.

12. Serve.

Prep Time: 15 Minutes

Cook Time: 45 Minutes

Servings: 2

Ingredients

- 1 tsp unsalted butter
- 1/4 cup onion (diced)
- 5 asparagus spears
- 2 large eggs
- 2 large egg whites
- 2 Tbsp water
- 4 Tbsp Parmigiano-Reggiano (grated)
- fresh ground black pepper (to taste)

Instructions

1. Preheat the oven to 400°F. Heat 1/2 teaspoon butter in a small non-stick sauté pan over low-medium heat and add the chopped onion. Cook until translucent and set aside. Slice the base of asparagus crosswise into small

rounds. Leave about 2 inches of the tops intact. Set the tops aside to decorate the top of the frittata. Whisk the eggs, egg whites and water in a bowl until frothy.

Heat the remaining butter in a small non-stick skillet over medium- high heat and when hot add the egg mixture. Reduce the heat to medium and simmer for about 2 minutes. At the end of one minute add the onion and chopped asparagus.

2. Arrange the asparagus tops in a star pattern on top of the cooking egg mixture. Scatter the parmesan cheese over the top and then fresh ground black pepper to taste.

Place in the oven. Reduce the heat to 350°F degrees and bake for 10 - 15 minutes until it puffs and is firm to the touch.

Prep Time: 15 Minutes

Cook Time: 45 Minutes

Servings: 2

Ingredients

- 1 tsp olive oil
- 1 small onion (diced)
- 1/2 large red bell pepper (diced)
- 12 ounces sweet potato (large dice)
- 1/4 tsp salt
- fresh ground black pepper (to taste)
- 2 tsp dried sage
- 2 large eggs
- 1 ounce reduced-fat Monterey jack cheese (grated)

Instructions

1. Preheat the oven to 375° F. Place the olive oil in a skillet over medium-high heat. Add the onions and sauté, stirring frequently, for about 2 minutes or until translucent.

Add the bell pepper and continue sautéing for another 2 minutes. Add the sweet potatoes, stir, and cover. Reduce heat to medium and cook for about 15 minutes, stirring frequently, until the potatoes are soft. Add the salt, pepper, and sage and stir. Cook for another 5 minutes on low.

2. Divide the potatoes between two oven proof dishes. Break one egg on top of the potatoes in each dish. Place the dishes in the oven and bake for about ten minutes until the eggs are almost done to your liking. Top with the grated cheese and bake for one minute or until the cheese is melted, then serve.

Prep Time: 15 Minutes

Cook Time: 45 Minutes

Servings: 2

Ingredients

- 2 tsp olive oil
- 1 medium eggplant (sliced horizontally into 4 thick rounds)
- 2 quarts water
- 1 Tbsp vinegar
- 4 large eggs
- 4 Tbsp Mustard Hollandaise Sauce
- 2 English muffins or gluten-free English muffins

Instructions

1. Place a large skillet in the oven and preheat oven to 325F.
2. Place 2 tsps olive oil in the skillet.
3. When oven comes to temperature, place the eggplant into the skillet, cut side down.

4. Roast for 15 minutes, then turn the eggplant over and roast for another 5 minutes. Remove the eggplant from the skillet and place the eggplant on a plate lined with a paper towel to cool. Set aside.

5. While the eggplant is roasting, make the Mustard Hollandaise per the recipe.

6. Keep the Hollandaise warm over very low heat, stirring occasionally. (See refrigerator light on this page.)

7. Place water over high heat and bring to a boil. Reduce heat to medium so the water is barely moving. Add the vinegar.

8. Crack each egg into a small dish or cup, taking care to keep the yolk whole. Add each egg to the poaching water and poach for 8-10 minutes.

9. While the eggs are poaching, toast the Engilsh muffins. Place a slice of roasted Eggplant onto each half of an English muffin. Remove the poached eggs from the water with a slotted spoon when ready to serve.

10. Top the eggplant with 1 poached egg and 1/4 sauce, then serve.

Prep Time: 15 Minutes

Cook Time: 30 Minutes

Servings: 6

Ingredients

- 1 large egg
- 2 Tbsp. reduced-fat spread
- 1/2 cup Splenda or stevia
- 2 Tbsp. non-fat yogurt
- 1/2 tsp. pure vanilla extract
- 1 cup all purpose flour
- 1/2 cup whole wheat flour
- 2 Tbsp. wheat germ
- 1/4 tsp. salt
- 1 tsp. baking powder
- 1/4 tsp. baking soda
- 1/2 cup low-fat buttermilk
- 1/2 cup blueberries

Instructions

1. Separate the egg into an egg white and egg yolk. Set the egg yolk aside and whisk the egg white until frothy. Add the reduced-fat spread and whisk together until smooth. Add the Splenda, egg yolk, yogurt and vanilla extract.

2. Whisk until smooth.

3. Place the all-purpose flour, whole wheat flour, wheat germ, salt, baking powder and baking soda in a sifter and sift into the mixing bowl.

4. Gently fold the creamed mixture together with the flour mixture. As this is blended slowly add the buttermilk folding until smooth. As soon as the mixture is well blended, stop.

5. Gently fold the blueberries into the batter. Do not over mix.

6. Line a muffin tin with 6 muffin papers and fill each muffin paper with an equal amount of batter. Bake for 12 – 15 minutes.

Prep Time: 15 Minutes

Cook Time: 30 Minutes

Servings: 6

Ingredients

- 2 lbs. bone-in, skin on chicken thighs (4 thighs)
- 1/2 tsp. salt
- 1/16 tsp ground white pepper
- 1/8 tsp ground black pepper
- 1/2 tsp ground mustard
- 1/2 tsp garlic powder
- 1 tsp paprika
- 1 tsp dried rosemary
- 1/4 tsp dried thyme
- 1/2 tsp dried marjoram
- 4 whole wheat or gluten-free hamburger buns
- 4 leaves butter or iceberg lettuce
- 4 slices fresh tomato

Instructions

1. If you are not able to find boneless, skin on chicken thighs, place the chicken thighs on a cutting board skin side down.

2. Using the tip of a boning knife, slice along the top of the thigh bone, slowly exposing the bone on either side but not cutting too deeply into the meat.

3. Gently separate the bone from the meat and reserve the bones for making chicken stock.

4. Place a large skillet in the oven and preheat the oven to 450F.

5. Place the salt, white pepper, black pepper, mustard, garlic powder, paprika, rosemary, thyme, and marjoram in a small bowl, blender, or mortar.

6. Using the back of a spoon, blender, or a pestle, grind the spices to powder.

7. Place the deboned thighs skin side down in a large bowl and sprinkle the spice mixture over the thighs.

8. Using tongs or your hands (wash your hands well before and after), turn the thighs several times to coat the thighs with the spices.

9. Place the thighs skin side down in the skillet and return the pan to the oven.

10. After 5 minutes, remove the pan from the oven, drain any fat from the pan, and using a spatula or tongs, press the thighs into the skillet to make sure the skin comes into full contact with the pan. Return the pan to the oven.

11. After another 5 minutes, repeat the draining of the fat and pressing of the thighs and return the pan to the oven.

12. After 2 minutes turn the thighs to skin side up and replace the pan in the oven.

13. Turn the heat to broil and broil for up to 5 minutes or until the skin is browned and crispy around the edges.

14. Do not overcook.

15. To serve, place each cooked chicken thigh on a bun and top with lettuce and tomato. Serve immediately.

Prep Time: 25 Minutes

Cook Time: 45 Minutes

Servings: 2

Ingredients

- 1 large red bell pepper
- 8 ounces boneless, skinless chicken thighs
- 1 tsp. chili powder
- 1 tsp. smoked paprika
- 1/4 tsp. ground cumin
- 1/8 tsp. cayenne pepper
- 1/4 tsp. salt
- 1 avocado (peeled and diced)
- 2 large green onions (thinly sliced crosswise)
- 6 corn tortillas or corn taco shells
- 1 Tbsp. fresh cilantro

Instructions

1. Preheat the oven to 350°F.

2. Place the pepper in the oven and roast, turning frequently, until it begins to blister on all sides.

3. Place the chicken thighs in a separate pan and place in the oven. Roast for about 12 to 15 minutes.

4. When the pepper is done, remove it from the oven and place in a brown paper bag, folding over the top.

5. Allow the pepper to cool for 10 minutes.

6. After the pepper is cool, peel and seed it and cut into 1/2 inch squares.

7. Once cooked, let the chicken cool and cut into 1/4 inch dice.

8. Place the diced chicken thighs in a bowl with the chili powder, paprika, cumin, cayenne pepper, salt, and avocado.

9. Chill well.

10. Serve the salad in the tortillas topped with the green onions and cilantro.

Prep Time: 25 Minutes

Cook Time: 60 Minutes

Servings: 8

Ingredients

- 1 Tbsp. olive oil
- 2 cloves garlic (minced)
- 1 medium onion (diced)
- 1/2 large red bell pepper (diced)
- 1 large rib celery (diced)
- 8 ounces mushrooms (minced)
- 1 – 15 ounce can no salt added tomato sauce
- 1 tsp. Worcestershire sauce
- 1/4 tsp. salt
- 1 1/2 tsp. dried basil
- 1 tsp. dried oregano
- 1/2 tsp. dried marjoram
- 1/4 tsp. dried thyme
- 16 oz whole wheat or gluten free spaghetti or linguine
- 8 ounces lentils
- 8 quarts water

Instructions

1. Place the olive oil in a large skillet over medium-high heat.
2. When the oil is hot add the garlic and cook for one minute. Stir frequently.
3. Add the onion and cook onions for 3 minutes. Stir frequently.
4. Add the pepper and celery and cook for 2 minutes. Stir frequently.
5. Add the mushrooms and cook for about 4 to 5 minutes. Stir frequently.
6. Add the tomato sauce, Worcestershire sauce, salt, basil, oregano, marjoram, thyme, and lentils.
7. Stir and cover.
8. Simmer for about 30 minutes over medium low heat. Stir occasionally. Add water 1/2 cup at a time if the sauce is too think.
9. Place the water in a large stock pot over high heat.
10. When the water boils, add the pasta and cook for about 12 to 15 minutes, until soft but still slightly firm.
11. Drain and serve the pasta with the sauce.

Prep Time: 25 Minutes

Cook Time: 60 Minutes

Servings: 2

Ingredients

- 4 medium poblano peppers
- 1 tsp. olive oil
- 1 medium white onion (minced)
- 1 small chipotle in adobo (finely minced)
- 3 ounces reduced-fat Monterey jack cheese (shredded)
- 4 Tbsp. fresh cilantro (coarsely chopped)
- 1 large egg
- 2 tsp. Dijon mustard (or chipotle paste)
- 4 ounces panko breadcrumbs or gluten-free panko breadcrumbs
- 1/4 tsp. ground cumin
- 1/2 tsp. smoked paprika
- 1/2 tsp. dried oregano
- fresh ground black pepper to taste

Instructions

1. Preheat oven to 350°F.
2. Place the poblano peppers in the oven and roast them for about 20 minutes.
3. Turn them about every 5 minutes: the skin of the chili should begin to turn black and soften.
4. Remove the peppers from the oven and place in a brown paper bag.
5. After about 30 minutes, the peppers should be cool.
6. Remove them from the paper bag and gently peel the thin skin from the pepper.
7. Using the point of a knife, cut around the stem end and gently remove the core and seeds from the inside, trying to keep the pepper whole.
8. While the peppers are roasting, place the olive oil in a large skillet and heat over medium high heat.
9. Add the onion and cook for 7 to 8 minutes.
10. Add the minced chipotle and cook for another two minutes.
11. Remove from the heat and chill the onion and chipotle mixture in the refrigerator for about an hour.
12. After the mixture is cool, toss it together with the cilantro and shredded cheese.

13. Form the resulting mixture into 4 small cylinders. Place the cylinders inside the peppers and reform the poblanos to resemble whole peppers.
14. Place the egg and mustard in a small bowl. Whisk until smooth.
15. In a bowl, place the breadcrumbs, ground cumin, paprika, oregano salt and black pepper. Mix together with a fork.
16. Preheat oven to 400°F.
17. Coat the peppers with the egg and mustard mixture and then coat with the seasoned breadcrumbs.
18. After all of the peppers are coated, place the peppers on a cookie sheet then put them into the oven.
19. Bake for about 7 minutes.
20. Spray lightly with spray oil and turn over, then cook another 7-8 minutes.
21. Serve immediately.

Prep Time: 25 Minutes

Cook Time: 30 Minutes

Servings: 2

Ingredients

- 1 cup water
- 1/2 cup quinoa
- 1 tsp. dark sesame oil
- 1/2 small red onion (finely diced)
- 4 cloves garlic (minced)
- 1/2 large red bell pepper (finely diced)
- 2 large green onions (thinly sliced crosswise)
- 1 tsp. lime zest
- 1/2 lime (juiced)
- 2 tsp. reduced sodium soy or tamari sauce
- black pepper to taste
- 8 large leaves bibb lettuce

Instructions

1. Place the water in a small sauce pan over high heat.

2. When the water boils, add the quinoa, stir, and reduce the heat to simmer.

3. Simmer the quinoa partially covered for 12 to 15 minutes until most of the water has boiled away.

4. Remove the pan from the heat, cover and let stand for 5 minutes.

5. Fluff the quinoa and transfer to the refrigerator to cool.

6. While the quinoa is cooking place the oil in a medium skillet over medium high heat.

7. Add the onion and garlic. Cook for 4 minutes. Stir frequently.

8. Place the onions in a mixing bowl with the red pepper, green onions, lime zest, lime juice, soy sauce and black pepper.

9. Add the cooked quinoa and toss well.

10. Chill well before serving.

11. Spoon the quinoa in individual lettuce leaves and top with Spicy Peanut Sauce.

DINNERS

21. French Onion Frittata

Prep Time: 25 Minutes

Cook Time: 30 Minutes

Servings: 2

Ingredients

- 1 whole wheat or gluten-free hamburger bun
- 2 tsp olive oil (divided)
- 1 large onion (sliced)
- 2 Tbsp no salt added vegetable stock
- 3 large eggs
- 2 Tbsp water
- 1 1/6 tsp salt
- fresh ground black pepper (to taste)
- 2 ounces provolone cheese

Instructions

1. Preheat the oven to 325°F.

2. Cut the hamburger bun into 3/4 inch chunks and place them on a cookie sheet.

3. Place the cookie sheet in the oven and toast the croutons for 10 minutes. Set aside.

4. Place a medium skillet over high heat.

5. Add 1 teaspoon olive oil, and when hot, add the onions. Cook the onions until caramelized: stir frequently and adjust the heat so that they don't burn.

6. When the onions are a caramel brown color, add the vegetable stock and cook for another two minutes until the liquid evaporates.

7. Remove the onions from the pan to a plate and let them cool for 10 minutes.

8. When they are cool, place the eggs, water, salt and pepper in a bowl and whisk until the eggs are frothy.

9. Add the onions to the bowl and fold them into the eggs until well blended.

10. Place a small skillet over high heat and add 1 teaspoon olive oil.

11. When the pan is hot, add the egg mixture and cook for about 30 seconds.

12. Place the pan in the oven and bake the frittata for about 10 minutes, until the eggs are almost set but the center of the top of the frittata is still slightly liquid.

13. Sprinkle the croutons over the frittata and top with the provolone cheese. Return the pan to the oven to bake for another 3 to 5 minutes, until the cheese is melted.

14. Serve.

Prep Time: 23 Minutes

Cook Time: 60 Minutes

Servings: 6

Ingredients

- 3 quarts water
- 1 1/2 lbs Yukon Gold potatoes
- 2 large red bell peppers
- 2 ounces prosciutto or Serrano ham (diced)
- 8 large eggs
- 1/4 cup 2% milk
- 1/4 tsp salt
- fresh ground black pepper (to taste)

Instructions

1. Place the water in a large stock pot over high heat.
2. Place the potatoes in the water and cook for about 45 minutes until a knife slips into the flesh with easily but with slight resistance.
3. Remove the potatoes and chill.

4. While the potatoes are cooking preheat the oven to broil.

5. Place a sheet of aluminum foil on the oven rack and put the peppers on top.

6. Roast until blackened turning to cook on all sides.

7. Remove and place in a paper bag to cool.

8. When cool, peel, seed, and cut into 1/2 inch squares.

9. When the potatoes are cool, cut them in half and then cut the halves into 1/4 inch sliices.

10. Preheat the oven to 325°F.

11. Place the eggs, milk, salt and pepper in a large mixing bowl.

12. Whisk until well blended and slightly frothy.

13. Pour about 1/2 cup into the bottom of a 10 inch Pyrex pie dish.

14. Add the ham and bell peppers to the egg mixture and whisk.

15. Place a single layer of potatoes in the bottom of the Pyrex dish.

16. Pour in half of the egg mixture.

17. Place another layer of potato slices.

18. Pour in the remaining egg mixture and then top with the final layer of potato slices.

19. Lightly pat the slices down so that the top layer is slightly submerged.
20. Place the tortilla in the oven and bake for 50 to 60 minutes.
21. Cool before serving.

Prep Time: 50 Minutes

Cook Time: 1hrs 30 Minutes

Servings: 4

Ingredients

- 1 quart water
- 1 large head cauliflower (broken into small flowerets)
- 1 tsp olive oil
- 1 large leek (sliced crosswise; keep white and green parts separate)
- 8 large eggs
- 4 ounces reduced fat cheddar cheese (grated)
- 1/4 tsp salt
- 1/8 tsp ground nutmeg

Instructions

1. Preheat the oven to 325°F.
2. Place the water in a large sauce pan fitted with a steamer basket over high heat.
3. When the water is boiling add the cauliflower.

4. Steam for about 10 minutes. Remove and let cool.

5. While the cauliflower is steaming place the olive oil in a medium skillet over medium high heat.

6. When the oil is hot add the white part of the leek and cook for about 2 minutes. Toss frequently.

7. Add the green part of the leek and cook for about 3 minutes. Toss frequently. Remove and let cool.

8. When the cauliflower is done, remove and let cool.

9. Place the eggs in a large bowl and whisk until frothy.

10. Add the cheese, salt and nutmeg.

11. Fold in the cooled leeks and cauliflower until well blended.

12. Place the mixture in a large pie pan or springform pan.

13. Bake for 60 minutes.

14. Serve.

Prep Time: 50 Minutes

Cook Time: 1hrs 30 Minutes

Servings: 4

Ingredients

- 2 tsp olive oil
- 1 large onion (diced)
- 16 ounces zucchini (cut into 1/4 inch dice)
- 8 large eggs
- 4 ounces provolone cheese (grated)
- 1/8 tsp salt
- 1/2 tsp dried basil
- 1/2 tsp dried oregano
- 1/4 tsp dried marjoram
- 1/4 tsp dried thyme leaves
- 6 large black olives (cut into slivers)
- 4 tsp capers

Instructions

1. Preheat the oven to 325°F.

2. Place 1 teaspoon of the olive oil in a medium skillet over medium high heat.
3. When the oil is hot, add the onion and cook for about 5 minutes. Toss frequently.
4. Remove and let cool.
5. Add the other teaspoon of olive oil to the pan and then the zucchini.
6. Cook for about 5 minutes. Toss frequently. Remove and let cool.
7. Place the eggs in a large bowl and whisk until frothy.
8. Add the cheese, salt, basil, oregano, marjoram, thyme, olives and capers. Whisk until blended.
9. Fold in the cooled onions and zucchini until well blended.
10. Place the mixture in a large pie pan or springform pan.
11. Bake for 40 minutes.
12. Serve.

Prep Time: 10 Minutes

Cook Time: 45 Minutes

Servings: 2

Ingredients

- 2 tsp. olive oil
- 1/2 lb. crimini mushrooms (sliced)
- 3 medium green onions (thinly sliced crosswise)
- 2 cloves garlic (minced)
- 4 large eggs
- 1/4 tsp. salt

Instructions

1. Place a small skillet in the oven and preheat the oven to 325°F.
2. When the oven is hot add the olive oil to the pan and swirl.
3. Add the mushrooms to the pan and return the skillet to the oven.

4. At five minutes toss the mushrooms in the pan and return the skillet to the oven.

5. At ten minutes add the garlic to the pan, toss well and return the skillet to the oven.

6. At fifteen minutes add the white part of the green onions to the pan, toss well and return the skillet to the oven.

7. Whisk the eggs until frothy. Add the green part of the green onions and the salt. Whisk.

8. At 20 minutes add the eggs to the pan, shake the pan gently, and return to the oven.

9. Bake for 10 minutes. Serve.

Prep Time: 10 Minutes

Cook Time: 60 Minutes

Servings: 6

Ingredients

- 2 1/2 lbs cauliflower (one large head)
- 4 cups water
- 2 tsp extra virgin olive oil
- 1 large leek (cleaned and thinly sliced crosswise)
- 5 cups water
- 2 ounces goat cheese
- 8 ounces reduced-fat white cheddar cheese (shredded)

Instructions

1. Cut the crowns from the stem of the cauliflower.
2. Divide into small flowerets and set aside.
3. Dice the stem.

4. Place the diced stems in a steamer and top with the flowerets.

5. Steam for 20 minutes and set aside to cool.

6. Place the olive oil in a medium stock-pot over medium-high heat and add the leeks.

7. Reduce the heat to medium and cook for 10 minutes. Stir frequently.

8. Add 5 cups water and half of the steamed cauliflower flowerets and the diced stem of the cauliflower.

9. Bring to a boil and reduce the heat to a simmer. Stir occasionally.

10. Simmer the soup for 30 minutes.

11. While the soup is simmering cut the remining flowerets into a small dice.

12. After 30 minutes remove the soup from the heat and let cool for about 10 minutes.

13. Using a blender or an immersion blender puree gently (the soup should have a bit of texture and not be completely smooth.

14. Return the soup to medium heat, and as it reheats, add the goat cheese and cheddar cheese and stir gently while the cheese melts.

15. Add the remaining finely chopped cauliflower flowerets and stir.

16. Heat gently on low for about 15 minutes and serve.

Prep Time: 50 Minutes

Cook Time: 1hrs 30 Minutes

Servings: 8

Ingredients

- 1 Tbsp. olive oil
- 2 medium white onion (diced)
- 2 cloves garlic (minced)
- 1 Lb. boneless chicken thighs (cut into 1/2 inch cubes)
- 3 – 15 ounce cans no salt added white beans
- 3 large russet potatoes (peeled and cubed)
- 2 cups vegetable or chicken stock
- 1/2 cup white wine
- 1 tsp. ground cumin
- 1 tsp. dried oregano
- 6 ounces reduced-fat white cheddar cheese (grated)
- 2 tsp. (per serving) non-fat sour cream
- 2 tsp. (per serving) reduced-fat white cheddar cheese (grated)
- 8 large green onions (thinly sliced crosswise)

- 2 avocados (thinly sliced)

Instructions

1. Place the oil in a large stock pot over medium heat.
2. Add the onion and garlic and cook for about 5 minutes. Stir frequently and don't let the onions brown.
3. Add the chicken and cook for about 5 minutes. Stir frequently.
4. When the chicken has browned lightly add the beans with the liquid from the can, potatoes, stock and white wine.
5. Add the cumin and oregano.
6. Stir and cook over low heat simmering for 60 minutes. Stir occasionally.
7. Add 4 ounces of the grated cheese, stir and heat through. Do not allow the chili to boil.
8. Serve with 2 teaspoons reduced fat sour cream, 1/4 ounce grated white cheddar, green onions, and 1/4 avocado per serving as garnish.

Prep Time: 15 Minutes

Cook Time: 45 Minutes

Servings: 2

Ingredients

- 1 orange
- 4 tsp. toasted sesame oil
- 4 tsp. reduced sodium soy or tamari sauce
- 1/8 tsp. fresh ground black pepper
- 1 Tbsp. fresh ginger root (peeled and finely minced)
- 1 Tbsp. minced parsley
- 3 Tbsp. black sesame seeds
- 2 - 4 ounce boneless chicken breasts (cut into 1 inch strips)
- spray olive oil
- 5 ounces baby spinach
- 2 small mandarin oranges or tangerines (peeled and sectioned)
- 1/2 medium red onion (sliced as thinly as possible)
- 3 Tbsp. slivered almonds

Instructions

1. Place a large skillet in the oven and preheat to 375°F.
2. Remove 1 teaspoon of orange zest from the orange and place in a blender or mini-chopper.
3. Juice the orange and add the juice to the blender with the soy sauce, pepper, ginger, and parsley.
4. Puree the dressing until smooth and place in the refrigerator to chill.
5. Preheat the oven to 425°F. Place a medium sized skillet in the oven.
6. Place the sesame seeds on a sheet of waxed paper.
7. Place the chicken strips one at a time in the sesame seeds to coat just one side of each strip.
8. Remove the hot pan from the oven and spray lightly with olive oil.
9. Place the chicken strips in the pan with the coated side down and return the pan to the oven.
10. After about 7 minutes turn the chicken strips over.
11. The chicken will take another 8 - 10 minutes to cook.
12. While the chicken is cooking place the spinach in a large bowl with the chilled dressing.
13. Toss until well coated.
14. Divide between two plates.

15. Sprinkle the mandarin oranges around the plate and then top with the almonds and sliced red onion.

16. When the chicken is done place the strips on top of the salad and serve.

Prep Time: 15 Minutes

Cook Time: 55 Minutes

Servings: 8

Ingredients

- 3 quarts water
- 2 lbs small red potatoes
- 1/4 cup reduced-fat mayonnaise
- 1/4 cup non-fat sour cream
- 1 Tbsp coarse ground mustard
- 2 Tbsp curley parsley (minced)
- 1/4 tsp salt
- 1/8 tsp fresh ground black pepper

Instructions

1. Place the water in a large stock pot fitted with a steamer basket.
2. Bring the water to a boil over medium-high heat.
3. Steam the potatoes for about 30 minutes until slightly soft.

4. Remove and let cool for about ten minutes and then chill thoroughly in the refrigerator.

5. Cut the potatoes into 1/2 to 1 inch pieces.

6. Place in mixing bowl and add mayonnaise, sour cream, mustard, parsley, salt and pepper.

7. Fold together gently and chill well before serving.

Prep Time: 15 Minutes

Cook Time: 60 Minutes

Servings: 4

Ingredients

2 cups 2% milk

1/2 cup non-fat dry milk powder

1 tsp pure vanilla extract

6 Tbsp Granulated Stevia

1/8 tsp salt

2 large egg yolks

8 tsp granulated sugar

Instructions

1. Place 2% milk, dry milk powder and vanilla extract in
    a medium sized non-reactive sauce pan. Heat over

medium heat until the mixture reaches 180°F. (This is the temperature that the milk will just begin to boil and at a higher temperature it will boil over.) Stir continuously and do not allow to boil.

2. Remove from the heat and allow to cool at least a few hours (preferably overnight in the refrigerator).

3. After the milk mixture is cool preheat the oven to 300°F. Fill a roasting pan with water to a level that will be about 3/4 of the way up a 1 cup ramekin. It is best to test this by placing the ramekins in the water bath to make sure it is not overfilled.

4. Place the roasting pan in the oven until the water is hot (this should take at least 20 minutes).

5. In a stainless bowl place the Splenda, egg yolks and salt. Cream together until smooth.

6. Strain the milk mixture through a fine sieve into the egg mixture. Whisk until well blended.

7. Divide the milk/egg mixture between four 1 cup ramekins. Place the ramekins in the water bath in the oven and cook for 60 minutes.

8. Very carefully remove the roasting pan from the oven and allow the custard to cool for 30 minutes while still in the water bath. Cover each custard with plastic wrap and chill overnight.

9. Place 2 teaspoons sugar on the top of each custard. Using a blowtorch melt the sugar by carefully aiming the tip of the flame at the surface of the sugar. Tilt and rotate the ramekin so that the melted sugar covers the surface of the custard. Serve.

10. Alternatively, the sugar can be melted under a broiler but the custard will need to cool again afterwards for about 10 minutes on the counter and another 20 minutes in the refrigerator.